ILEOSTOMY DIET COOKBOOK

A Comprehensive Guide For Both Beginners And Pro-Nourishing Recipes, Meal Plans, Expert Guidance And Pro Tips For Optimal Digestive Health And Vitality

DR. JACE ZAYDEN

Table Of Contents

Copyright © 2024, Dr. Jace Zayden

All Rights Reserved

No part of this publication may be reproduced, distributed, or transmitted in any form or by any means, including photocopying, recording, or other electronic or mechanical methods, without the prior written permission of the publisher, except in the case of brief quotations embodied in critical reviews and certain other noncommercial uses permitted by copyright law.

DISCLAIMER

The information provided in the book is intended for general informational purposes only. The content of this book should not be considered a substitute for professional medical advice, diagnosis, or treatment.

Readers are advised to consult with a qualified healthcare professional for medical advice tailored to their individual circumstances.

The author has made every effort to ensure that the information in this book is accurate and up-to-date at the time of publication. However, medical knowledge is constantly evolving, and new research may emerge that could impact the information presented. The author disclaims any responsibility for any adverse effects or consequences resulting from the use of the information provided in this book.

References or mentions of individuals, products, websites, organizations, or other names within this book are for informational purposes only and do not constitute an endorsement. The author has no affiliations with, and makes no endorsements of, any third-party entities mentioned. Readers are encouraged to conduct their own research and exercise their judgment when considering any external resources or recommendations.

The author and the publisher shall have neither liability nor responsibility to any person or entity with respect to any loss, damage, or injury caused or alleged to be caused directly or indirectly by the information contained in this book. Any reliance on the information within this book is at the reader's own risk.

By reading this book, the reader acknowledges and agrees to the terms of this disclaimer. If the reader does not agree with these terms, they should not use the information provided in this book.

ABOUT THIS BOOK

This book entitled "Ileostomy Diet Cookbook" is an all-encompassing manual that functions as an indispensable supply for those who are adjusting to life after undergoing an ileostomy. The introductory segment establishes the context by providing a comprehensive explanation of the essential elements of ileostomy, thereby facilitating comprehension of the surgical process and its ramifications. Acknowledging the utmost significance of a specialized diet in the period following surgery, this book provides readers with practical advice on how to effectively manage their nutritional requirements during this critical time by meticulously outlining immediate dietary guidelines.

An aspect that sets this book apart is its methodical structure, which progressively assists readers as they encounter foods that are appropriate for an ileostomy diet. The articulation of which foods should be consumed and which should be excluded becomes an essential resource for those in search of dietary clarity. The inclusion of nutritional supplement exploration and hydration management as focal points enhances the discourse, providing readers with the knowledge necessary to make well-informed dietary choices.

Advice on meal planning, techniques for managing digestive difficulties, and guidance on diet monitoring and adjustment collectively offer a comprehensive viewpoint on maintaining a healthy lifestyle following ileostomy surgery. The incorporation of expert guidance highlights the publication's dedication to providing readers with access to authoritative opinions. Additionally, lifestyle factors are taken into account, recognizing the wider ramifications of an ileostomy on one's day-to-day existence.

In addition to providing theoretical understanding, this book also offers practical support through a dedicated section that includes recipes and meal ideas specifically designed for individuals who have undergone an ileostomy. This book provides a systematic response to frequently inquired concerns regarding the ileostomy diet, thereby serving as a convenient reference for readers in need of immediate clarification.

This "Ileostomy Diet Cookbook" serves as an essential resource, providing individuals navigating the challenges of living with an ileostomy with information, practicable approachable strategies, and a sense of empowerment. By its extensive subject matter, this book serves as a dependable companion, encouraging well-informed judgment and facilitating a more seamless progression towards a harmonious and satisfying post-ileostomy way of life.

CHAPTER ONE

ILEOSTOMY DIET: BEYOND SURGICAL NOURISHMENT FOR LIFE

Introduction

Ileostomy surgery is a transformative experience that necessitates substantial physical and emotional adaptations. An ileostomy is a surgical procedure in which a portion of the small intestine is brought to the surface through the creation of an orifice in the abdomen called a stoma.

This aperture functions as a waste escape, circumventing the colon and rectum. Those who undertake this procedure frequently encounter difficulties acclimating to their altered lifestyle and dietary habits.

A critical element of life after ileostomy is the implementation of a specialized diet that promotes holistic well-being while addressing the distinct challenges associated with ileostomy care.

Comprehension Of Ileostomy

Before delving into the complexities of an ileostomy diet, it is critical to grasp the physiological transformations that occur as a consequence of the operation. As the organ responsible for nutrient assimilation, the small intestine is crucial to digestion. By performing an ileostomy, the digestive process is redirected, circumventing the colon, which is the primary site of water absorption. As a consequence, stoma output is increased in frequency and liquid consistency relative to regular bowel movements.

Having an ileostomy necessitates adjusting to a modified digestive process. The material expelled through the stoma is devoid of the water absorption that is characteristic of the colon; thus, nutrient absorption and hydration become critical concerns. Furthermore, specific food items have the potential to affect the regularity and consistency of bowel movements, thereby potentially disrupting the quality of life for individuals with ileostomy.

For this reason, it is crucial to adopt a customized approach to nutrition to preserve health and avert complications.

The Critical Role Of A Specialized Diet

In addition to facilitating physical adaptation to the post-operative changes, a specialized ileostomy diet is vital for preventing complications and maintaining optimal health. Dehydration is a significant concern for individuals who have undergone ileostomy. Elevated levels of fluid in the discharge may result in electrolyte imbalances; therefore, a diet abundant in fluids and electrolytes is crucial.

Additionally, particular dietary selections may have an effect on the consistency of feces, which in turn may affect the frequency of ostomy bag changes and the overall level of comfort experienced. Foods that have the potential to induce flatulence, emit odors, or obstruct should be handled with extreme caution. A nuanced comprehension of one's body and a willingness to experiment with various foods to identify personal triggers are necessary for managing these factors.

Regarding ileostomy diets, there is no universal method. The process entails customizing food selections by personal preferences, dietary restrictions, and tolerance levels. Seeking guidance from a registered dietitian or healthcare professional who specializes in post-ileostomy nutrition is of the utmost importance when it comes to formulating an individualized dietary regimen that addresses lifestyle and medical considerations.

Prompt Post-Surgical Dietary Directives

Ileostomy patients must prioritize the period immediately following surgery, during which the body heals and adjusts to the surgical modifications. In this stage, dietary decisions are of the utmost importance in facilitating recovery and averting complications. Frequently, it is recommended that patients begin on a low-fiber diet to facilitate digestion.

Vegetables that are prepared thoroughly, lean proteins, and refined grains are examples of foods that are easily digestible and reduce the likelihood of blockages or irritation.

Over the course of recovery, individuals may reintroduce fiber into their diet in a gradual manner. Soluble fibers, which are present in cooked vegetables, cereals, and bananas, are generally more well-tolerated by individuals as they supply essential bulk without inducing excessive flatulence or discomfort. It is advisable to proceed with caution when introducing insoluble fibers, which are found in nuts, seeds, unprocessed fruits, and vegetables, as they have the potential to increase feces output.

Hydration is of the utmost importance immediately following surgery. Adequate fluid consumption aids in the prevention of dehydration, promotes recovery, and preserves electrolyte balance. Urine color monitoring is an uncomplicated yet efficacious method of verifying adequate hydration; a delicate yellow hue signifies the consumption of sufficient fluids.

Apart from dietary considerations, it is imperative for individuals who have an ileostomy to prioritize their general health. Sustained adherence to healthcare recommendations regarding physical activity, maintenance of a healthy body weight, and prompt resolution of any concerns are all factors that contribute to an effective recovery.

In summary, managing daily life with an ileostomy necessitates not only physical adaptation to a modified anatomical structure but also a deliberate and knowledgeable approach to nutrition. A specialized ileostomy diet plays a pivotal role in enhancing overall quality of life, preventing complications, and promoting health. By gaining knowledge of the distinct gastrointestinal obstacles that arise after undergoing surgery and following individualized dietary recommendations, patients can initiate a process of fortitude and wellness that extends beyond the limitations of their surgical procedure.

The Ileostomy Diet: A Guide To Achieving Wellness

It is possible for ileostomy living to be a life-altering experience, in which patients must adjust to a new way of life. Surgically, an ileostomy is performed by creating a stoma, or orifice in the abdomen, through which excrement is redirected to an external pouch. Dietary modifications are frequently required to accommodate this disruption in the digestive system to maintain optimal health and well-being. This article will provide an in-depth analysis of critical elements of the ileostomy diet, encompassing the methodical incorporation of foods, inclusion and exclusion of specific foods, and fluid management.

A Methodical Approach To Gesturing Following Surgical Procedures

After undergoing ileostomy surgery, it is critical to reintroduce foods into your diet with extreme caution and gradually. It takes time for the digestive system to recover; therefore, consuming an assortment of foods at once could potentially overburden it and result in complications. It is essential to begin with low-fiber, readily digestible foods and progressively increase the complexity of your diet.

Commence by consuming bland foods, such as white rice, basic pasta, and thoroughly cooked vegetables that have been stripped of their coverings. These commodities are hypoallergenic and aid in the detection of particular triggers or intolerances. You may gradually reintroduce lean proteins such as fish or chicken as your body adapts. Maintaining a food diary during this period is recommended to monitor one's body's reaction to various foods, thereby enabling well-informed decision-making regarding personal preferences. A progressive increase in fiber consumption is recommended, as an excess of fiber can lead to abdominal discomfort and an increased frequency of digestive movements. Consider consuming cooked vegetables and fruits such as pears and avocados, which contain soluble fibers. With caution, incorporate insoluble fibers, which are present in whole cereals and unprocessed vegetables, into one's diet, as they may in certain instances cause blockages.

Incorporating Foods Into An Ileostomy Diet: Sustaining Body Well-Being

The process of developing a dietary regimen for individuals with an ileostomy entails the careful selection of foods that not only supply vital nutrients but also exhibit minimal impact on the digestive system. A variety of nutrient-dense foods should be prioritized to supply the body with essential vitamins and minerals.

1. Incorporate lean protein sources, such as tofu, poultry, turkey, fish, and eggs, into your dietary regimen. These substances supply vital amino acids that are necessary for the repair of tissues and overall well-being.

2. Select low-fiber fruits and vegetables, such as peeled apples, avocados, and well-cooked vegetables that retain their coverings. These options provide vital nutrients and minerals while avoiding superfluous weight gain.

3. To begin with, opt for refined cereals such as white bread, white rice, and bland pasta, as they are more easily assimilated. As your tolerance improves, progressively incorporate whole cereals into your diet, such as whole wheat products and brown rice.

4. Low-lactose or lactose-free dairy products should be incorporated into the diet to prevent potential digestive issues. Yogurt and lactose-free milk are both viable options for obtaining calcium.

5. Incorporate healthful lipids into your diet in moderation, such as avocados, olive oil, and nut butter. These factors enhance overall vitality and well-being.

6. Maintain proper hydration by consuming sufficient fluids, such as electrolyte-rich beverages and water, to avert dehydration. Adequate hydration is of the utmost importance to preserve electrolyte equilibrium, particularly in light of the augmented fluid loss via the stoma.

CHAPTER TWO

Foods To Prevent: Mitigating Potential Difficulties

Certain foods should be avoided when constructing a nutritious diet after having an ileostomy to prevent distress and complications. While there may be individual variation, the following general principles can be beneficial:

1. It is advisable to restrict the consumption of high-fiber foods, such as unprocessed fruits and vegetables, nuts, seeds, and whole cereals, due to the potential for increased bowel movements and blockages.

2. It is advisable to restrict the consumption of gas-producing foods, including legumes, cabbage, broccoli, and carbonated beverages, due to their potential to induce congestion and heightened gas production.

3. It is advisable to limit the intake of piquant and irritant foods, as they have the potential to induce

inflammation and cause adverse effects on the digestive system.

4. Particular Fruits and Vegetables: Exercise caution when consuming foods that contain fibrous components, seeds, tough coverings, or other tough portions of particular fruits and vegetables.

Managing Fluid Intake: Maintaining Optimal Hydration For Health

Ensuring adequate fluid balance is of utmost importance for patients who have an ileostomy. Increased fluid loss through the stoma may result in dehydration and electrolyte imbalances. The following are some recommendations for the management of fluid intake:

1. Staying Hydrated: It is crucial to consume a sufficient quantity of water throughout the day. Water facilitates digestion and prevents dehydration.

2. Electrolyte-Rich Beverages: To restore electrolytes depleted due to increased bowel

movements, incorporate electrolyte-rich beverages into the diet, such as sports drinks or oral rehydration solutions.

3. Caffeine and alcohol should be consumed in moderation, as they have the potential to cause dehydration. Choose decaffeinated or water-infused beverages instead.

4. Observe Urine Color: Observe the hue of your urine; adequate hydration is indicated by a mild yellow hue, whereas dehydration may be indicated by a dark yellow hue.

In summary, maintaining a balanced ileostomy diet necessitates a deliberate and incremental approach to reintroducing foods, selecting alternatives that are abundant in nutrients, circumventing potential obstacles, and regulating fluid consumption. It is recommended to seek guidance from a healthcare professional or a registered dietitian who specializes in ostomy care to customize dietary recommendations according to specific dietary requirements and tolerances.

By adopting a mindful dietary approach, individuals who have undergone ileostomy can optimize their general health and effectively traverse the trajectory towards a gratifying and disease-free existence.

Supplemental Nutritional Supplement Navigation

Adherence to a restricted diet is essential for individuals with an ileostomy to maintain optimal health and well-being. An ileostomy is a surgical procedure involving the creation of a stoma, an orifice in the abdomen that facilitates the expulsion of feces into a pouch. Adequate nutrition is critical for individuals who have undergone ileostomy to sustain energy levels, promote recovery, and avert potential complications. The use of nutritional supplements is essential to reaching these objectives.

Individuals who have an ileostomy encounter the possibility of experiencing nutrient deficiencies as a result of compromised digestion and absorption.

During the operation, the small intestine, which is the primary site of nutrient assimilation, is either bypassed or partially removed. This hurts the body's capacity to extract vital vitamins and minerals from food. As a consequence, dietary supplements are an advantageous component of the ileostomy diet.

B vitamins, vitamin D, and calcium are frequently depleted in ileostomy patients. Deficiencies in calcium and vitamin D, which are vital for healthy bones, can result in complications such as osteoporosis. Folic acid and B vitamins, such as B12, are indispensable for energy production and cell division. The provision of these nutrients as a supplement aids in bridging the lacuna caused by the altered digestive process.

Furthermore, supplemental nutrition may be required due to the increased fluid and nutrient loss caused by the use of a high-output ileostomy pouch. Electrolytes, including sodium and potassium, are essential for supporting nerve and muscle function and maintaining fluid balance.

Potential imbalances can be mitigated through the consumption of electrolyte-rich foods and the incorporation of electrolyte supplements.

Collaborating closely with healthcare professionals, including dietitians or nutritionists, is crucial for individuals with an ileostomy to ascertain their specific supplement requirements. Periodic blood tests might be advised to monitor nutrient concentrations and make necessary adjustments to supplement dosages. It is essential to strike a balance, as overconsumption of supplements can result in its own set of health complications.

In essence, nutritional supplements serve a crucial function in promoting the well-being of individuals undergoing ileostomy by mitigating the risk of possible deficiencies in essential nutrients. A personalized approach is achieved through collaboration with healthcare professionals, which assists individuals in maintaining optimal nutritional status and overall well-being.

Tips For Effective Meal Planning On The Ileostomy Diet

Individuals with an ileostomy must adhere to a nutritious and balanced diet to facilitate the healing process, avert complications, and uphold general health. Meal planning assumes a pivotal role in the daily routine, aiding in the management of digestive obstacles and the optimization of nutrient consumption. The following are some effective meal-planning suggestions for ileostomy patients:

1. It is crucial to maintain proper hydration by consuming sufficient fluids to prevent dehydration, particularly in cases where the ileostomy results in increased output. Hydration can be maintained with the aid of electrolyte-rich beverages, water, and medicinal remedies.

2. Fiber management may be necessary for individuals with an ileostomy, who, despite the general recommendation for digestive health, should consume a high-fiber diet, and must consider their personal fiber tolerance. Generally,

soluble fibers, which are present in cereals, fruits, and vegetables, are more tolerable than insoluble fibers.

3. Constraint Your Meals to Three: Instead of consuming three substantial meals throughout the day, opt for smaller, more frequent meals. This can aid in ileostomy output volume management and discomfort prevention.

4. Eating and Mindful Chewing: To facilitate digestion, chew food thoroughly, and consume slowly to enable the body to efficiently process and assimilate nutrients. This may also decrease the likelihood of stoma obstruction.

5. Achieve a balanced nutrient intake by incorporating an assortment of essential nutrients into your diet. Prioritize the consumption of lean proteins, whole cereals, fruits, and vegetables to obtain vital vitamins and minerals.

6. Restrict Gas-Producing Foods: Certain food items, including cabbage, legumes, and carbonated beverages, have the potential to

induce gas production. A moderation and monitoring of these substances' consumption can aid in the alleviation of discomfort.

7. Maintain a food diary to identify particular foods that have the potential to induce digestive distress or stimulate an increase in bowel movement. This data can guide individualized meal preparation.

8. Investigate Food Texture Varieties: to determine food preferences and intolerances, conduct experiments with various food textures. Cooked or pureed foods may be more easily digestible for some individuals.

9. It is advisable to seek the advice of a registered dietitian or another healthcare professional who specializes in providing nutritional support for individuals with an ileostomy. They are capable of offering customized guidance to certain individuals' preferences and requirements.

10. Supplement as Necessary: As directed by healthcare professionals, incorporate nutritional

supplements to address potential nutrient deficiencies.

Meal planning for individuals undergoing ileostomy ultimately necessitates a synergy of cognizance, trial and error, and cooperation with healthcare practitioners. Through the utilization of well-informed decision-making and dietary customization to suit individual requirements, people can maximize their nutritional consumption and experience a state of wellness and contentment in their lives.

CHAPTER THREE

Overcoming Digestive Obstacles

Ileostomy-related difficulties are especially pronounced in terms of digestive health. Digestion and nutrient assimilation may be impaired as a result of surgically altered anatomy, necessitating the development of coping mechanisms to ensure a comfortable and satisfying existence. The following are some suggestions for managing the digestive difficulties that accompany an ileostomy:

1. Engage in the practice of mindful dining by meticulously chewing food and deriving pleasure from every mouthful. This may facilitate digestion and decrease the likelihood of stoma obstruction.

2. Adequate fluid consumption should be maintained to prevent dehydration, particularly in cases where the ileostomy produces an increased volume of fluid. Beneficial are water, herbal infusions, and electrolyte-rich beverages.

3. A well-balanced diet is one in which a variety of nutrients are consumed. Vegetables, fruits, lean proteins, and whole cereals all contribute to digestive health as a whole.

4. Fiber Management: Adapt fiber consumption by individual tolerance. Generally, soluble fibers, which are present in foods such as cereals and avocados, are more tolerable than insoluble fibers.

5. Gas-Producing Foods: To mitigate discomfort, restrict the consumption of foods that induce gas, including cabbage, legumes, and carbonated beverages.

6. Maintain a food diary to identify particular foods that have the potential to induce digestive distress or stimulate an increase in bowel movement. Dietary modifications can be guided by this information.

7. Investigate Food Texture Varieties: to determine food preferences and intolerances, conduct experiments with various food textures.

Certain people may discover that foods that are milder or liquefied are more easily assimilated.

8. It is advisable to consume smaller, more frequent meals throughout the day to regulate the amount of fluid expelled from the ileostomy and mitigate any potential discomfort.

9. Consider integrating probiotics into your dietary regimen as a means to foster a harmonious equilibrium of intestinal microbiota. Healthcare professionals should be consulted for individualized recommendations.

10. Supplementation: Collaborate with healthcare practitioners to ascertain whether nutritional supplements are necessary to compensate for possible deficiencies in essential nutrients.

11. Emotional Support: Consult mental health professionals, healthcare professionals, or support organizations for emotional support. Navigating digestive difficulties can impose significant emotional strain, underscoring the criticality of having a support network.

12. Consistent Check-ups: Establish a routine for consultations with healthcare practitioners to assess general well-being and promptly attend to any developing concerns.

13. Adherence to appropriate stoma care protocols is crucial for preserving hygiene and averting infections. An appropriately maintained stoma is beneficial for the digestive system as a whole.

14. Embrace lifestyle modifications and adjust routine activities accordingly to accommodate the ileostomy. Being well-organized and ready can assist in mitigating the tension and anxiety associated with digestive difficulties.

15. Maintain knowledge regarding ileostomy maintenance and digestive health. Acquiring knowledge enables individuals to exercise autonomy in decision-making and advocate for their welfare.

Managing digestive difficulties after ileostomy necessitates a comprehensive strategy encompassing dietary modifications, lifestyle adaptations, and emotional assistance. By taking proactive measures to confront these obstacles, individuals can achieve personal fulfillment while efficiently navigating the repercussions of an ileostomy on their digestive well-being.

Dietary Monitoring And Adjustment For Ileostomy

Dietary monitoring and adjustment is an essential component of ileostomy management. Due to the potential for nutrient deficiencies and altered digestive anatomy, a proactive approach is required to ensure optimal health. Key factors to bear in mind when monitoring and modifying the diet are as follows:

1. Consistent Monitoring: Establish a routine for consultations with healthcare practitioners, such as nutritionists or dietitians, to assess one's nutritional status and overall well-being. Nutrient levels may be evaluated through the utilization of blood assays.

2. It is imperative to maintain a state of constant vigilance to identify any indications of nutrient deficiencies, including but not limited to fatigue, frailty, and alterations in the skin and hair. Detection at an early stage enables timely intervention.

3. Personalized Dietary Plans: Foster partnerships with healthcare professionals to formulate individualized dietary plans that effectively cater to specific requirements, while also considering potential obstacles in nutrient absorption.

4. It is advisable to periodically reevaluate the necessity of nutritional supplements and make any required adjustments to the dosages. Healthcare professionals can make more informed recommendations with the aid of blood tests.

5. Vigilant hydration monitoring is essential, particularly in situations where the ileostomy results in an elevated discharge of fluids. As

dehydration may be an issue, it is vital to maintain adequate hydration levels.

6. Maintaining a comprehensive food diary serves the purpose of monitoring dietary patterns, identifying foods that cause digestive difficulties, and identifying trigger foods. This information may serve as a guide for dietary adjustments.

7. Implementing a flexible meal planning strategy entails making necessary adjustments to food selections by individual reactions to various cuisines. Self-awareness and experimentation are crucial in determining what works best.

8. Collaborating with Experts: Sustain transparent lines of communication with healthcare practitioners to deliberate on any modifications in digestion processes, energy levels, or general state of health. Immediate dietary modifications can effectively avert complications.

9. Monitoring Stoma Function: Maintain vigilance regarding the stoma's function,

encompassing aspects such as discharge consistency, color, and dimensions. Potential matters that necessitate attention may be unveiled by alterations.

10. Sustaining the practice of mindful dining with an emphasis on gradual consumption and thorough chewing is recommended. Eating mindfully facilitates digestion and decreases the likelihood of stoma blockages.

11. Gradual Introductions: To assess the potential impact of novel foods on digestion, it is advisable to introduce them progressively. This facilitates the identification of potential stimuli and enables a more regulated process of adjustment.

12. Proactive Approach to Difficulties: Adopt a proactive stance when confronted with digestive challenges. Immediately consult with healthcare professionals for advice, and be prepared to make any required dietary modifications.

13. Maintain a comprehensive understanding of educational resources about ileostomy care and dietary management. Knowing enables people to take an active role in managing their health and overall well-being.

14. Adaptation to Lifestyle Changes: Acknowledge the potential for dietary requirements to undergo modifications over time and demonstrate a readiness to accommodate these shifts. Long-term well-being may be enhanced by implementing lifestyle modifications.

15. Emotional Wellness: Recognize the psychological ramifications associated with ileostomy care and its potential to affect dietary patterns. When necessary, seek emotional support to preserve a positive outlook.

Dietary monitoring and modification following ileostomy is a dynamic process requiring continuous collaboration with healthcare professionals.

By maintaining a proactive stance and exercising informed judgment, individuals can maximize the benefits of their dietary selections, bolster their general well-being, and elevate their standard of living.

CHAPTER FOUR

Application For Expert Opinion

It is imperative to consult healthcare professionals, specifically a registered dietitian or a nutritionist with expertise in the management of patients with ostomies, after undergoing an ileostomy. Personalized guidance can be rendered by these specialists on an individual's unique lifestyle, medical condition, and nutritional requirements. Dehydration, nutrient deficiencies, and weight management are a few of the potential obstacles associated with an ileostomy that may be addressed in a balanced diet with their assistance.

It is imperative to seek professional guidance when Customizing Your Diet to Manage Potential Complications. For example, dehydration may result from increased fluid and electrolyte loss in certain individuals who have undergone ileostomy. A dietitian may suggest incorporating water-rich foods into one's diet and imbibing electrolyte-rich beverages as methods to maintain adequate hydration.

Additionally, dietary modifications may be required to mitigate the risk of obstructions or irritation in the vicinity of the stoma. The selection of foods that are readily digestible and less prone to causing discomfort can be assisted by a professional.

Consistent follow-ups with a healthcare team can guarantee continuous support and facilitate necessary dietary adjustments.

Lifestyle Factors To Consider:

As you adjust to life with an ileostomy, there are lifestyle factors to consider that may influence your dietary decisions. A healthy and vigorous lifestyle must be maintained with consideration for its prospective effects on the digestive system. Consistent physical activity can facilitate digestion, enhance general health, and assist in stress management, all of which may be exacerbated during the period of adjustment.

It is particularly important to plan regarding meals and hydration. It is advantageous to bring along a water bottle and munchies, as this will guarantee that you remain adequately hydrated and nourished throughout the day. Furthermore, possessing knowledge regarding the whereabouts of public restrooms can offer reassurance and mitigate potential apprehensions regarding the management of one's ostomy while traveling.

Additionally, emotional health is a crucial component of lifestyle choices. Obtaining counseling or participating in support groups can assist you in managing the emotional difficulties that accompany having an ostomy. A constructive perspective and a community that provides support can substantially enhance one's quality of life.

Meal Plans And Recipes:

A balanced and pleasurable dietary regimen is essential for sustaining optimal health and contentment with one's meals.

The following are meal suggestions and general guidelines for individuals with an ileostomy:

Favor milder, properly prepared foods to facilitate the process of digestion. Tender proteins, cooked vegetables, and pureed potatoes are all viable options.

• Maintain proper hydration by consuming water in small amounts throughout the day. Caffeine and alcohol should be avoided in excess, as they may exacerbate dehydration.

• Fiber Intake: Reintroduce fiber into your diet gradually to support digestive health. Commence with dietary fiber sources that are readily digestible, such as fruits and vegetables that have been thoroughly cooked and stripped of their coverings.

• Protein Sources: Maintain a sufficient protein intake to support tissue repair and promote overall health. One may incorporate plant-based proteins, lean meats, eggs, and dairy into their diet.

• Small, Regular Meals: To mitigate digestive burden and avert potential discomfort, opt for smaller, more frequent meals throughout the day as opposed to large meals.

• Consume foods abundant in fluids: To promote hydration, integrate soups, stews, and smoothies into one's diet.

Frequent Questions Regarding The Ileostomy Diet:

Can I consume my preferred foods while carrying an ileostomy?

A: Yes, in many instances. Nevertheless, it is imperative to systematically incorporate them into your routine while closely observing your body's reaction.

Certain foods may induce irritation or discomfort; therefore, it is critical to exercise caution and modify one's diet accordingly.

How can methane and odor associated with an ileostomy be managed?

A: Conduct experiments involving various cuisines to identify those that might be a contributing factor to heightened gas production. In addition, the implementation of odor-neutralizing products, adequate hydration, and proper pouching techniques can aid in the management of these issues.

Can alcohol be consumed while having an ileostomy?

A: Although moderate alcohol consumption is generally deemed acceptable for individuals with ileostomies, it is crucial to closely observe the physiological response of one's body.

Alcohol can cause dehydration; therefore, it is essential to increase water consumption in addition to alcohol consumption.

Are there any foods that I ought to entirely abstain from? A:

The effects of particular nutrients differ between individuals. Still, unprocessed vegetables, seeds, legumes, and foods high in fiber are frequently encountered as problematic. It is prudent to progressively incorporate these foods into your diet while monitoring your body's reaction.

In summary, the effective management of an ileostomy necessitates a comprehensive strategy encompassing consulting experts, taking into account lifestyle variables, examining a variety of meal plans and recipes, and responding to frequently requested inquiries. By receiving appropriate assistance and knowledge, people who have ileostomies can lead gratifying lives and consume a nutritious and balanced diet.

Conclusion

In conclusion, individuals who have an ileostomy must acquire and adhere to a balanced ileostomy diet to preserve their quality of life and overall health. Managing digestive symptoms, preventing dehydration, and ensuring adequate nutrient assimilation are the principal objectives of this diet.

Maintaining a balanced fiber intake is crucial to prevent potential obstructions. To determine one's tolerance levels, individuals should systematically reintroduce specific foods. Hydration is of the utmost importance, particularly in light of the increased fluid loss through the stoma. To aid digestion, it is recommended to distribute meals throughout the day in smaller, more frequent portions.

Although specific food restrictions are common on the ileostomy diet, for personalized guidance, it is vital to consult with healthcare professionals or a registered dietitian. With their knowledge, individuals can customize their diet to address particular requirements, taking into account variables such as age, physical condition, and way of life.

In essence, a proficiently administered ileostomy diet enables individuals to experience a sense of satisfaction in their lives by facilitating ideal nutrition and reducing the likelihood of potential complications.

The success of this dietary approach is contingent upon education, continuous support, and consistent communication with healthcare providers. These factors empower individuals to adopt a healthy and well-balanced lifestyle following ileostomy surgery.

THE END